PRA

"I devoured in one sitting this upbeat, profound, inspirational guide to a richer, fuller life with the gusto and guts that Nancy alone could bring to this topic. I've already started my 4-week program by rereading the book and I am on the path to more freedom and play as of today."
~ Dr. Diane Sukiennik, *The Career Fitness Program: Exercising Your Options*

"Nancy B. has written a book that shares her God-given gift of an elevated level of common sense and down-to-earth wisdom. It is a powerful book that can't be rushed through, or read just one time. Rather it is a manual to be kept by the bedside and referred to every day."
~ Patricia Pierson, *I Have Your Little Girl, The Runaway Widow*

"Nancy Berggren's new book is a fresh, irreverent look at how to lead a passionate, fulfilling life at any age – especially as we grow older. She cuts through stereotypes of how we 'should' age and presents a mode of living life to its fullest with grace, gratitude, and generosity. Her book is a powerhouse packed with punches left and right and is definitely worth a read."
~ Dr. Michael Reiss, Educator, Consultant

"Nancy B. has done it again. Written a book that is perfect for me and for anyone who wants to live their best life AT ANY AGE. It is practical, filled with tips to focus our attention. It is personal, coming from her authentic self that lets me trust and try it out. Then it is provocative with her juicy questions--- simple yet compelling. You can tell from the cover that being perky and playful is as important as being self-aware and kind to ourselves."
~ Dr. Barbara Leger, Co-Founder & Inspirational Officer, Golden Path of Peace

"I was deeply moved by Nancy's book. She is a pioneer of a spirituality that defies rules, shifting from life advice to life practice, transcending ages. It draws from the splendor of ancient wisdom, but has been entirely reimagined to become tangible medicine for our time. Nancy imparts a spiritual truth often forgotten: Age is never just a matter of numbers but rather a state of mind."
~ Michel Pascal, *Meditations for Daily Stress*

Books by Nancy B. Berggren

Life is a Game and You Can Play It
Spinning Mistakes into Gold, Gathered by Marilyn Miller
(contributing author)

To HELL With Aging!

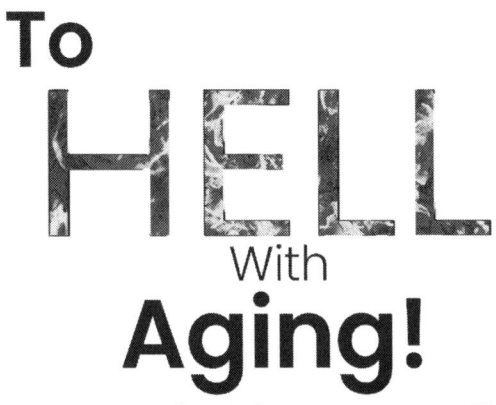

7 Lessons for Living an Ageless Life

Nancy B. Berggren

Copyright © 2024 by Nancy B. Berggren

All rights reserved.

No portion of this book may be reproduced in any form without written permission from the publisher or author, except as permitted by U.S. copyright law.

To My Family,
Who Fill My Heart With Joy and Gratitude,
To My Faith-filled, Fun-Loving Friends and
All Who Walk this Beautiful Road Home with me.

"When you feel love in your heart,
you are calm and at peace, and all rebellion
leaves you."
~ White Eagle, *The Beautiful Road Home*

Contents

Foreword	XIII
Introduction	1
1. What's On Your Mind?	7
2. Do One Thing	17
3. Use It or Lose It	25
4. Grace and Gratitude	35
5. Feeling Sad, Lonely, Depressed, Scared?	43
6. Love Life, Love Others	53
7. Want More Intimacy, Love, and Sex?	59
8. Your Turn: Take Action	69
Acknowledgements	75
Books That Changed My Life	77
About the Author	79

Foreword

7 Lessons for Living an Ageless Life
by
Dr. James Mellon

They say that the perfect teacher comes into your life when you, the student, are ready. Well, I can see that. I can also see that the perfect book comes into your life when you, the reader, are ready. I think that's what is happening with this book you are about to enter. I say enter, because it's more like a playground for your soul than words on a page, or chapters in a book. More to the point, the woman who wrote this powerful exercise in breaking the rules of aging, is a powerful force for transformation in this world. Those who encounter her "energy" are never the same. Trust me, I'm one of those people.

I met Nancy "B," as she is affectionately called by those who know her, when she was merely in her 70's. She was the picture of health, vibrancy, mischief, spontaneity, and unbridled joy and excitement. She was trying to blend into the congregation of my Spiritual Center and not call much attention to herself. By her own words she had retired from ministry and was now in a "laying low" state of mind. Well, trying to lay low for Nancy B is like taking a flashlight into a dark room, turning it on and then expecting no one to notice. WE ALL NOTICED! And before you knew it, she was an active force in the forward trajectory of all we were doing. Nancy gave retirement a whole new meaning. She branded it in such a way that all of us wanted to be like that woman at the other table in "When Happy Met Sally," who pointed to Meg Ryan and said, "I'll have what she's having." We wanted what Nancy knew, and more to the point, we wanted her kind of ageless youth and vitality at any age.

I dare say that the book you have before you is a gift that you will be so glad you gave to yourself. And if someone else gave it to you, even better. You are clearly loved. The inimitable force that is Nancy B is something of an enigma. Watching her live her life and reading what is behind the consciousness that has lived it, are sometimes very different things.

She is so honest here in terms of letting the reader in on her process, that she makes us all feel as if we are reading our own lives out loud. We may not have done stand up comedy at 80, but we've taken risks and pivoted in our own lives enough times that we get what she's telling us. And how beautifully and caringly she lets us in. It's as if she's narrating our own personal lives and we get to sit back and realize just how amazing we are.

The wonderfully irreverent Rev. Nancy Berggren has written a book that illustrates 7 lessons for living an ageless life. If I were you, and I am, I would pay attention and try these lessons out. Take them for a ride. You just might find something that has been there all along that is time for you to let loose ... at any age.

~ Dr. James Mellon, *Mental Muscle, The 5 Questions*

Introduction

"There's a naked man in my bed!"

That was the first line in the stand-up comedy routine I did at the Comedy Store on Sunset Boulevard in Hollywood in my 80's! As an actor, I was boring and bored. I decided to do something that would shake me up; that would force me out of the safety of the 'box' I had gotten so comfortable with! When I asked myself what that was, I answered, 'Stand-Up Comedy.'

It was a great success. I got a standing ovation, but when they asked me to come back, I thought, no way Jose! If I had any doubts, the guy before me who did a seven-minute routine on his proctology exam with a rubber glove on his hand finished me!

I wrote this book because, perhaps unlike you, I've been a people pleaser and a perfectionist most of my life. It was tough for me to do anything I felt I was so far outside of the box, that I would be disapproved of. Needless to say not everyone was thrilled with my departure into stand-up comedy. But I did it and I am still totally amazed and proud of myself.

What scares you that you've always wanted to do?

What is your secret dream? What would happen if you did it? Who is going to disapprove, your mother? What are you longing to do, but were always afraid to try? What is it: hot air ballooning, wind surfing or sky diving? How about pole dancing? Go ahead. You know you always wanted to do it. Just don't hurt yourself. In five years, you'll still be five years older, whether you do it or not.

I wrote this book because we're making it up as we go along. None of us have been here before. I have no idea what it's like to be a 91 year old woman who feels more like 70.

Let's all have more fun in our Golden Years and let them be the best years of our lives. You can do it and so can I. So here we go!

Yes, I know you want to skip to the Chapter 7, *Want More Intimacy, Love, and Sex?* so go ahead. I wrote it for you, so enjoy! When you're done, come on back and let's see what kind of mischief we can get into together.

ONE MORE SONG TO SING
Music and Lyrics by Nancy B. Berggren

The kids say come home mama,
The grandkids miss your face.
You really ought to slow down now,
And we fixed you up a really nice place.

But I can't come home right now kids.
I've got some things to do.
You see my books a best seller, I met a new feller,
We're off to Tim-buck-tu, woo, woo, woo.

I cut my hair and dyed it too,
I'm wearin' a size three,
And if you wanna' see your mama kids,
Just turn on your TV.

No, I can't come home right now kids,
I got some bells to ring.
And before I walk that long, long road,
I've got one more song to sing

So don't you put me out to pasture,
Lock up that Granny flat.
This Grandma's learnin' Salsa,
'Cause that's where the actions at. Ole!

I can't come home right now kids,
I got some bells to ring.
And before I walk that long, long road,
I got one more song to sing.

Now I know you think I'm old kids.
Sure came as a surprise to me.
So sing your songs and ring your bells,
'Cause someday, you'll be me, and you'll say,

I can't come home right now kids,
I got some things to do.
I got mountains to climb, rivers to cross,
See all my dreams come true.

I'm layin' down this heavy load,
I still got some gifts to bring.
I got one more mountain, a few more dreams,
and one more song to sing.

Chapter 1
What's On Your Mind?

> "There is a Thinking Stuff from which all things are made and which, in its original state, permeates, penetrates, and fills the interspaces of the Universe."
> ~ Wallace Wattles, *The Science of Getting Rich*

Wow! Heavy stuff! But it's exciting too, because it means that right where you are, right now, this very moment, this Thinking Stuff is, in all its fullness. It is ready and willing to do your bidding. It is malleable, fluid, plastic. It receives your thoughts and acts to bring them into form. It has no ideas or desires of its own. It is the servant of *your* thoughts and beliefs. It is the engine in your Prius or BMW; powerful, but inert until you, the driver, tell it where you want to go. Sometimes, I've noticed that I am asking for, or claiming one thing, but believing something else. What are you believing?

I believe and expect to be able to dance at 91, so I dance. I believe and expect to still drive my car, so I drive and it's not a big deal. However, I don't believe, or expect that I can sleep through the night without sleep aids, so I can't. *My beliefs make it so*. I can shout to the rooftops all day long that I can do it, but if my deeply held belief says I can't, it silently trumps my want or desire, no matter how loudly I shout. Your subconscious beliefs are often running the show totally without your awareness.

That's what's happening when something you've yearned for and worked toward for so long continues to be delayed. Ask yourself if there could be something in your belief system that is denying it. You are worthy of receiving the riches of the Universe, but what it gives *To* you, it can only give *Through* you. Your conscious awareness of this Truth can be the beginning of a exciting new adventure. You can live the life of your dreams, with the partner of your dreams, in the home of your dreams, but only if you *Believe you can* and have nothing left in your subconscious mind that denies it.

Your mind is part of this Thinking Stuff. It is not separate from you, something you need to go in search of. It has been with you, working through you all the time, with or without your knowing. What an awakening it can be to know that you can work in harmony with this Infinite Source to bring about the desires of your heart! The following is a statement of truth I created years ago.

Since the One Mind is all Knowing and everywhere present, all my needs are known and provided for instantly and constantly by my own Inner Source of Limitless Supply.

My *'Inner Source of Limitless Supply'* is this Thinking Stuff, or the One Mind! If it can make oceans and babies and bees and trees, hang stars in the sky and provide food for seven billion of us every day, it can certainly create the perfect home, with the perfect housemates for me. And it's easy. A piece of cake! In fact that is its major function, but if I don't give it clear, specific instruction, I may get a messy, mixed up version of my desire. The following is my messy example.

My daughter-in-law agreed to drive me to the airport. I was going to visit my son and his wife in Gardnerville, Nevada and was excited and eager to get going. So excited that I brought my carry-on to the garage in advance so I'd be ready to go when she picked me up. I got in the car with my water bottle, jacket, boarding pass, purse etc. while she put the luggage in the car. When we got to the airport, she stood my snazzy blue and orange suitcase up on the sidewalk and said, "This will be easy." I replied, "Yes, I'll just put the other piece on top." She asked "What other piece?" Yep! You got it. The 'other piece' was sitting in the garage right where I put it!!!!!

Obviously, I wasn't specific. When I said luggage, I meant two pieces, but she only saw one. I didn't ask if she got both pieces, I took it for granted. My bad. We flew back down the freeway, grabbed it, and flew back to the airport. Somehow, by the grace of God, we made it.

If you tell your spouse you're hungry and want them to bring you something to eat for dinner, don't throw a fit when he/she brings you Hot Wings or Sushi if you don't eat them. If you want Alfredo Pasta with sun-dried tomatoes and mushrooms, ask for that. Be specific. Do no less when dealing with the Thinking Stuff, this One Mind.

The Thinking Stuff is listening to your thoughts *all the time*, not just when you are praying about something you want to create or change. It's the thoughts *in between*, in your car, in the shower, in your bed before sleep, that can get in the way, if you're not paying attention.

> *"Once you know that everything in your life arises from consciousness, you start looking pretty closely at what goes on between your ears. Change that and you change your*

world."
~ Marianne Williamson, *The Gift of Change,*

I had repainted the master bedroom preparing to welcome a new housemate to my home. I put an ad in Craigslist, created an affirmation, stating that they were already there, living in the space and that we were all blessed by this perfect, new individual. But they did not come! Months went by as I got more frustrated and upset at my inability to *make this happen.* I was counting on this extra income and it just wasn't happening. What did I do wrong? Oops! Notice what snuck in there when I wasn't looking? We can't *make* anything happen! We can *cooperate* with the infinite givingness of the Universe and *allow* a greater good to come into our lives. When we try to get our way, in our time, we are getting in the way of the natural flow of the Divine circuits, whose only desire is to give us good things.

Life is a Flow, constantly moving and changing and we need to be willing to allow it to reveal our perfect next step, which may be entirely different, or better than what we originally had in mind. Have you ever failed to manifest something you thought you really wanted, only to discover that, had you gotten it, you wouldn't have been available for a Much Greater Good, the Universe had in store for you? I have. When we understand how the Universe works, when we acknowledge its continuous action in our lives and give thanks for it, we are in the flow and things seem to unfold magically right before our eyes.

One Sunday, I said out loud to my deceased husband, 'I need to make an appointment with you tomorrow.' He was the steady, quiet thinker, and was the catalyst that I needed to move out of trying to control this situation out of fear and being stuck! I knew it was something in me, in my subconscious mind, or belief system that was keeping it from me. It had to be, because the Universe always says Yes!

On Monday morning, I sat down in my meditation chair with his picture and a journal to capture the thoughts as they arose. I sat there, sometimes talking, sometimes shutting up and just listening, or writing in my journal for two and a half hours. I refused to get up until I felt at peace in my heart, knowing and trusting the Universe to bring me exactly what I needed, exactly when I needed it. When I felt totally at peace, I gave thanks for the much-needed opportunity to clear my head. When I stood up, I heard "It all goes fast now." At 8:00 AM the next morning, I got a text from the Perfect Person, the one we'd been waiting for. He was an absolute delight. I couldn't have written it any better.

Tip#1: The Universe works perfectly every time, everywhere, in all things, as all things. It never denies you, it doesn't know how, even if your desire is not for your highest good. If it's not working for you, you are the only one who might, unconsciously, be blocking the flow.

Tip #2: Check your consciousness, your beliefs. Are you trusting the Universe to know what you need and to supply it, or are you fearful that it won't happen? Any hidden fears will block the natural flow.

A Course in Miracles says there are only two emotions: Love and Fear. If you're not feeling the emotion of love — open and trusting, however it expresses itself — they say you are in fear. Love expands, opening the way for your good to come to you. Fear contracts, sometimes closing that door to your good.

Tip #3: When you know what you want, write a positive affirmation, declaring that it's already yours! Use the most powerful, expressive words you can and keep it in the Now. Remember, you are acting as if you are already living your dream!

Tip #4: Your Feelings are the key. Notice when you are really pissed off, how much energy you put out. That same level of energy needs to be present when you speak your statement of truth aloud, morning and night!

How thrilled you will be when that new Mazda or Audi shows up in your driveway, or the promotion and huge raise comes through, or the lover of your dreams walks into your office. Let yourself Feel it Now. That will help to pave the way for it to come to you.

Tip #5: End your statement by expressing your Joy and Gratitude for the blessings in your life *before they arrive*. That is the second key.

Example: This is the positive affirmation I wrote for my new home when I was moving from Oceanside to Santa Clarita.

> *My perfect new home is light-filled and spacious, with a welcoming air of warmth and elegance. It is surrounded by magnificent park-like grounds. I feel totally safe here, am gloriously happy and deeply grateful.*

Notice a couple of things. When you read it, you can *feel* my passion, my joy and gratitude, all before I had even found it! Notice too that I didn't describe the physical structure. I talked about how gloriously happy I would *Feel* when I was actually living in the home of my dreams.

When I went out with the real estate agent, I was disappointed in what I saw, but I kept saying my affirmation with joy and gratitude all day long, believing and knowing that the Universe already had my perfect home picked out for me. All I had to do was stay positive, Expecting to receive it.... and I did. It was so perfect that tears of gratitude came to my eyes.

Your Turn: Write your Gratitude *As If* you have already Received it and are Living your Dream Now! If you are reading a digital copy, grab your journal and write your Affirmation there.

I am So Grateful that .... (and then write what you are grateful for)

OK, you know what to do, but nobody can do it for you. Think big, but keep it real. Imagine that you are living your dream. Picture yourself with that perfect person, in that environment, living and loving your life. Let your heart swell with gratitude for the blessings you have received and those that are on their way. Times a wasting! So do it now.

Chapter 2
Do One Thing

When you keep your word with the Universe, the Universe keeps its promise to you. It always says, "Yes!"

When I moved to Santa Clarita from Oceanside in 2004, I didn't know a soul except for my young son's family. But they worked, taught their four girls homeschooling and weren't available most of the time. So I thought, I need to do something to get out and meet people!

I signed up at the local community college. I took performing arts classes, (back to my first love). Today, some Community Colleges in California are actually *free* for the first two years! Wow! Check it out. No excuse for me not to sign up! I was 71 years old.

The first week in school I was cast in a musical, Big River. We opened the Santa Clarita Performing Arts Center. From that I was cast in an independent, film, *Outpost*, which we shot in the desert in the summer heat near Palmdale. I was off and running, doing what I loved.

That's when a divine happening occurred. A manager, Fran Blain saw me in class at the Ruskin Theatre in Santa Monica and signed me up. For the next ten years, with her rooting for me, I had the opportunity to work with people like Jim Carrey, Zach Galifinakis, Frank Langella, and Placido Domingo in an LA Opera at the Music Center.

Tip #1: Here is one of the best things I've learned in the last 40 years. It is fail safe. It's like a proven scientific principle. Like your favorite recipe for Red Velvet cake. Follow the recipe and you get perfect cake *every time*! So here it is. Drum Roll please!

Do One Thing Every Day toward your Goal

You can't fool the Universe. When you really commit and leave no escape route open in case you want to quit, the Universe will move too. It will bring to you exactly what you need exactly when you need it. Miraculous Serendipities occur. The right people show up at the right time, venues appear out of nowhere. A casual conversation at your favorite coffee shop with someone who accidently spilled their iced venti in your lap leads to opportunities beyond your wildest dreams! Once you've begun, and see the benefits you've received, you would never want to quit! Why would you?

Remember this though. All this took place because you were doing the work every day to reach your goal. Believe me, nothing comes from doing nothing. I know because I tried it, more than once. Sitting at home waiting for the phone to ring won't bring you what you want.

That's it. Pretty simple. Every time I used it consistently, I got work! Every time! If it's so simple, and it always produces results, and it did, why wouldn't everyone use it all the time?

Did you ever try to stop smoking, or give up sugar or alcohol, or to exercise daily, or lose weight or whatever? You started out with a clear intention. You'd read the research, you knew it was the right life choice for you and you made a decision that you were going to do this!!!

How long did you last? A week, a month? What stopped you? No judgment, just notice. Become an observer of your own life. With the best of intentions, life gets in the way. One of the kids, or you, gets sick. Covid hits, or the IRS decides to audit you. Your lover or spouse walks out, and on and on. Life happens.

Tip #2: *Your Dream has come true* and you are movin' and groovin', enjoying it all. It's beyond your wildest dreams and you're feeling like all things are possible! Watch out for sneaky little interrupters that may try to knock you off course. Take a moment and think back to all the time and energy, the consistent dedication it took to get you there. You don't even notice as your daily practice begins to slip to ten minutes... when you remember... until it stops all together. It's easy to forget the effort it took for you to get that far. Rededicate yourself to staying focused on what you want, coupled with gratitude for Knowing it's your conscious cooperation with the 'Thinking Stuff' that brought it about.

Tip #3: It takes tremendous discipline coupled with desire to stick to your plan. It feels like the moment you make the decision, the Universe says, "Oh, this ought to be fun. Let's see how fast I can break this one up." But that's not what's happening. It's just the daily demands of living life on this planet; the distractions, the urgent needs of family or friends. It is also an opportunity for you to be on the look-out for sneaky little intruders whispering in your ear, "It's too late, and your sooo tired. (Boo Hoo) Let's go sit down and have a beer, or a Klondike bar. You can do that other thing tomorrow." But tomorrow becomes another today, and round and round you go.

Tip #4: If your dream seems overwhelming and you don't know how to begin, chop it up into bite sized chunks. *Your Book Now* writing coach, Thor Challgren, told us about how CNN news anchor, Jake Tapper, successfully wrote and published two novels, by writing just 15 minutes a day! If he can do it with his demanding schedule and family needs, we too can find 15 minutes a day to pursue our dreams. Here is something I found absolutely magical when I wanted to write my first book, but had no idea how to do it.

Try this. On a piece of posterboard, create a staircase. Make the steps wide enough so that you can write on each one. I like to take time and make it pretty with colored pens etc., but that's up to you. At the top, sketch a picture of your dream. This is not an art project (although it can be). Just make it so you know what it means. At the bottom, draw a stick figure of you. Now you should have 15 or so steps to help you reach your dream. Start at the bottom and write one thing you can do each day to keep moving toward your goal.

Tip #5: They don't have to be big; but they have to be real. They just have to keep your heart and head consciously involved in thinking about your dream, your goal, on a daily basis.

Tip #6: Here's a way to back up your staircase sketch. If you live in a two-story house, you can use each step to remind yourself that you are moving confidently and expectantly toward your goal. Each time you go upstairs, say or think:

I move step by step toward my goal

And what about escalators? All you need to do is take the first step and the Universe does the rest! You have a silent Partner who is always ready to provide the way once you decide where you want to go. Move with energy and enthusiasm.

You might want to sell your house and move to be closer to your kids, or downsize. You might want to buy a car, swim with the dolphins in Florida, or take a cruise through the Panama Canal. All those things take planning. As we age, we need to take special care to make sure all our bases are covered before we take off. Here are some ideas to get you started.

Tip #7: Make a list of all the possible actions you can think of. As you actively work with your list, more inspired ideas will come to mind. Add them to your list.

DO ONE THING 23

Research someone who did what you want to do. Find out how they did it.

Call someone you would never think of calling and ask them for their help. Make notes about the *specific points* you want to cover. The clearer and more specific you are, the more they will likely feel inspired to help you.

Write a positive statement about your goal. What is its purpose? How will it work? How will it benefit others? How will it be funded, if necessary?

If needed in your plan, write a resume, or update the one you did in 2017. You know what to do, so get to *Play*!

Notice I didn't say 'get to work.' I did it for a reason. When you approach a new project with excitement and enthusiasm, you are working in harmony with the attributes of the Universe: Peace, Love, Joy, Harmony, Wisdom, Beauty, Abundance, Health, Wholeness and more. Don't call it work, even in your mind. Call it Play, make it easy and decide you will have Fun doing it.

Remember, when you make a commitment and stick to it, the Universe moves too. It will bring together all you need to make your dream come true. Notice it usually comes step by step, (Aha! Our staircase) not all in one chunk. The Universe wants you to succeed, so that It can be more fully expressed in form. It all starts with an idea, a dream, from the field of Infinite possibility. Refer to Chapter One, *What's On Your Mind?*, for more on the subject of how it works.

Chapter 3

Use It or Lose It

"Eat Well, Sleep Well, and Exercise."
~ Esther Jones, RScP Emeritus

As our bodies age, their functions may slow down. Eating like you did as a teenager or young adult: pizza and beer, fries, a Big Mac, and a shake may, over time, leave you feeling unwell.

My dear friend Esther says when things feel out of control, and nothing is working, she goes back to what she can control: eat well, sleep well and exercise.

During a prolonged illness last year, I lost weight. Always super slim like my family, losing weight was not a plus. I prayed nonstop asking for clarity and guidance. Tried every suggestion from family and friends, and changed my diet. Meanwhile my back broke out in a nasty rash that continued to spread; itching, bleeding, and making me miserable.

After dermatologist visits, and applying every cream on the market, I was getting desperate. One morning in a dreamy, half-awake state, I clearly heard *"Sugar is poisoning my body."* Pretty clear and the one question I never asked, *because I didn't want to hear the answer*! Could that be what was causing my back to break out? If so, I needed to listen up and make a change.

Sugar is addicting. More so than cocaine they say. And I was addicted. Yuck! I didn't want to go cold turkey, so I made an agreement with myself to have *one sweet a day* and it's working, most of the time. You might want to try it. Sometimes I slip, then I remember to love myself back to peace. I remind myself that all I have to do is *change my mind and think a new thought!* How hard could that be?

I also had to stop hating this itching, bleeding mess on my back and embrace, love and appreciate my body, just the way it was! The energy we put into hating any part of ourselves, comes back to bite us in the rear. More about this later.

Your body is miraculous! It functions nonstop to give you the energy you need to do what you came here to do! It makes fingernails, toes, elbows and hair out of the Alfredo

Pasta with mushrooms and sun-dried tomatoes you had for dinner last night. You don't know how it does that and most of the time aren't even aware of the process, which goes on 24/7. Life is living you. When you decide to cooperate with it, wanting a healthier body, ask for guidance. It will show you, in some mysterious way, exactly what you need and do not need.

Tip #1: Is there something about your body, your finances, or your relationships that you *secretly* hate? The more you hate it, the more deeply entrenched it becomes. Why? Because *what you focus on expands.* We live in a *cause-and-effect world.* What you put out comes back. Give love, and live a love-filled life. Give the *opposite of love* and you'll find yourself surrounded by that as well. For example, with the sores on my back, *the more I hated it the more it spread.*

I invite you to exchange the energy of hate for the energy of love. Even if you don't feel like it. Even if you don't believe it, do it anyway. Make it an experiment, an adventure and have FUN with it. What if this simple step could release the misery you've held onto in any area of your life? Are you willing, or do you still have to be Right? If you find yourself struggling to let it go, ask to be willing to be willing. Lighten up!

> "The secret to enjoying life is to take an interest in it."
> ~ Thomas Troward

Are you enjoying your life, just the way it is? Do you want it to be better? Do you want to be happier? Ask yourself honestly if there is anything you are holding onto that you need to let go of. You may be amazed at the energy and joy of living that shows up when you have released it! I was. It was there all the time. Just clouded over by the messiness of my negative thinking.

When you get clear about what it is you really want, when you declare it and stick to it, it will show up. It may take a while, or show up today. Either way, you're the winner and beneficiary of a happier, healthier life.

<u>Tip #2</u>: Stop Complaining! Stop talking about your messy, sad, unfair, awful situation to anyone who will listen! Because now you know that:

> The more Energy, or Attention you give it...
> the more it will expand!

Ask yourself if that is what you really want? If not, make an agreement to *catch yourself* when you start to complain. Be ready and willing to trade that thought for the next better feeling thought. Do not make yourself wrong. You are learning a new way to live a happier, more fulfilling life. Chances are you probably won't do it perfectly every time. I certainly didn't and that's OK. You are moving in a positive direction.

> Congratulate yourself for every time you remember and let go of the times you forget.

I'm embarrassed to admit that *I did exactly what I am advising you Not to do!* That's how I figured out *It didn't Work!* Yep! My itchy, yukky breakout became my #1 topic of conversation! (boring!) I also insisted on *Showing it* to those poor souls who hadn't made their escape. When they said, 'That's not so bad.' I corrected them immediately by saying *"Oh yes, it is! It's awful! I Can't sleep! I've tried everything and nothing works!"*

Can you hear me *Fighting For* the very thing I so desperately wanted to get rid of? It was definitely *not* something I wanted *more of*. It's hard to see, insidious and sneaky, when we're in the middle of it. Problems, challenges, situations that need our attention may come our way. Having a clear, calm mind aids us in finding solutions. If you feel stuck and need help, ask someone who always speaks a higher Truth for you when you can't see it for yourself. Remember a time when you helped a friend through a sticky situation and know someone out there is willing and eager to help you too. Let yourself be vulnerable and willing to change. You, like me, will be so grateful when you are on the other side of it and can look back and realize the wisdom you gained and the steps you took that got you there.

> Now I need to Congratulate myself for
> the times I remembered and Let Go of the
> times I forgot!

I struggled with sleepless nights for years; wandering the house in darkness, wondering how much longer it would be before the sun came up and I could sleep. There is tons of information out there to help us overcome this malady. Here are a couple of things I've learned that have helped me enjoy sleeping well again.

Tip #3: Never watch CNN or a scary movie and then go to bed. Your subconscious mind will replay all night long the fear, anger, or pain you felt while watching it. Instead, begin turning the lights down, quiet your mind and body. You might play some soft, meditative music while you get ready for bed. My favorites are on *Yellow Brick Cinema* on YouTube. Just type in *Meditation Relax Music*, then scroll down and pick your favorite.

Tip #4: This is my *Favorite New Thing* and it works like a charm for me! When you are finished with your evening ritual; the doors are locked, the lights are out, any animals are taken care of, try this. Have a favorite book; a novel or inspiring reading on your nightstand. Climb into bed and read a chapter or two. When your eyes get heavy, without any disturbance, lay your book down, turn off the lamp and snuggle down into your cozy bed. You are peaceful and relaxed. As you close your eyes, breathe a silent prayer of thanksgiving for another blessed day of life.

If you need more help with your sleep habits, talk to your doctor. I did that and tried everything out there without success. Then a friend recommended Sleep Gummies with CBD. Hallelujah! Blessed Uninterrupted SLEEP! They work like a charm for me. Most nights I sleep straight through till morning, not even getting up to pee! Always check with your doctor if you are on medications to make certain sleep aids are safe for you before beginning to take them. Also, use a reputable CBD pharmacy. You can order gummies through Amazon, but since I am a new user, I prefer to talk to a knowledgeable, trained person who can guide me to the best product for me.

Tip #5: Walking is still number one for me. I write more about it in Chapter Five, *Feeling Sad, Lonely, Depressed, Scared?* But for now, know how valuable walking can be. Next to swimming, walking is the best exercise for your body. It's easy and it's free. I walk twice a day. In the morning, sometime before 12:00 noon, I walk a mile or so around my neighborhood. There is always so much to see: how the roses are blooming up and down the street, how the fruit is ripening on the orange, lemon, plum, fig and pomegranate trees. All bathed in the sweet glow of a beautiful new sunny, or windy, or cool day. In the evenings, I look forward to the sunsets that grace me with their ever-changing colors and beauty.

Tip #6: Check out Dr. Zach Bush *4 Minute Workout* on YouTube. I love it. It exercises your whole body in such a short amount of time. He also explains the benefits to your body from a medical point of view. I just know that it works. At 83 years old, I established it as a regular part of my daily routine. And guess what? I discovered muscles in my flabby arms which had totally forgotten what a muscle was!

Tip #7: If you've had an injury to your body, or are recovering from surgery, look for a water exercise class. The YMCA has programs designed specifically for this kind of recovery. I was so grateful that I found them when I was recovering from a painful back injury.

From Random Acts of Love, author unknown, here is a thought you might want to tuck away in your phone so you can refer to it in the future.

Eat like you love yourself,
Move like you love yourself,
Speak like you love yourself,
Act like you love yourself.
Love yourself.

Chapter 4
Grace and Gratitude

"Gratitude is the gateway through which
more blessings flow."
~ My Mother

Your neighbor's dog continues to poop on your grass, the IRS is withholding your refund, your water heater broke and water is seeping onto your practically new carpet. The more upset you get, the more fuel you throw on the fire, escalating it out of proportion. Your gut tightens, your stomach churns and a headache begins to throb.

You want to yell at somebody or throw something. But you can't because you are a civilized person, and it's not ok to yell or throw things. But your gut is still churning and your headache is becoming more painful by the moment. What to do?

Many years ago, I got into a dispute with AT&T. I don't remember the issue. I think they were charging me some exorbitant fee for a mistake they made and were trying to put it off on me. We went back-and-forth for weeks. I cried. I beat my chest. I tore my hair out (figuratively speaking). I stomped my feet and the mess got worse and worse. (Feeding the flames.)

I finally had to sit myself down and give myself a good old talking to. I knew better. I knew how cause-and-effect worked. I knew that what I put out, I got back in spades. I could see that all the anger, rage, and bitterness I was pouring out, I was definitely getting back. But how to change it?

I had to *forgive myself* for losing it big time, (I did kind of yell) and realize the person I was speaking to was just doing her job. It had nothing to do with her. I needed to come from a place of love and gratitude. Gratitude for the service they provided and love for the people who did their best to provide it. I had to release it all and begin again, because it still wasn't resolved. Once I really let it go, it was all settled quickly, easily and effortlessly. But how could someone actually do that? What steps could you take?

Tip #1: Back off. Take a breath. Sit down alone, if you can, and just breathe. Relax. You might journal about your *feelings*. Is there a bigger issue at work here? Is something going on beneath the surface? Ask yourself what that might be? When in the past did something similar occur, perhaps in childhood? Did you feel unseen or unheard? Were your thoughts and feelings ignored or disrespected? Breathe and let that scared little kid reveal its fears to you. Let it cry if it needs to. Reassure it that you are here now, and will never allow it to be disrespected or unheard again.

Take another breath. Exhale slowly. Sit quietly for a few minutes. Be grateful for the truth that was revealed and healed. Take another breath. Notice if all the angst, the tension in body and mind have begun to dissipate and are disappearing. Be glad. You might even smile and hug yourself for the good work you are doing. In a year from now chances are you won't even remember the incident or if you do, you will probably laugh at it.

Just the other day I caught myself replaying an old tape in my head about something super upsetting that happened when I was *10 years old*! I laughed out loud and said, "What are you doing? That was healed and released ages ago." Then I was able to let it go and move on.

Tip #2: Laugh at yourself. At the nonsense you get yourself into. Lighten Up! When you can laugh at yourself, it releases the pent-up energy around the issue, whatever it may be, clearing the way for a new, lighter, brighter understanding or point of view.

> "Everything you're against weakens you.
> Everything you're for empowers you."
> ~ Wayne Dyer, *The Power of Intention*

Nothing weighs down your heart and robs you of your joy more than unforgiveness. It becomes a dark cloud, blocking out the sun, that freely offers its warmth, wisdom, and light to guide you on your way. Stumbling in the dark, you bump into others who, like you, can't figure out how they got there.

Ta-Da! Drum Roll! It doesn't matter how you got there! All that matters is, are you going to continue looking down into the pit of misplaced self-righteousness, or are you ready to look up into the light of forgiveness that releases you from the prison of unhappiness that you created with your thoughts. Because *Thoughts become Things*. Read more about that in Chapter One, *What's On Your Mind?*

If you find your busy, ego mind grousing about your neighbor, or your kids, or your in-laws, or the government, you might use Jose Silva's suggestion in *Silva Mind Control* and say, *Cancel-Cancel* with energy! You may have to say it several times until you feel the energy release. Then replace it with something positive. Ask yourself, What am I most grateful for in this very moment? It could be as simple as: There's food in the fridge, gas in my car and money in my wallet. I'm good. Write in your journal what you are most grateful for in this moment.

Tip #3: Grace allows you to acknowledge and say "I've made mistakes too; I've said and done hurtful things I wish I could take back, but I can't. What I can do is release this one I've held in bondage for so long, so that we can both be free!" The jailer is just as stuck in prison as the one he or she is guarding.

Ho'oponopono is an Ancient Hawaiian prayer of forgiveness. It translates simply as, *'making things right.'* See if it resonates with you. You can use it to make amends for any hurt you may have caused, known or unknown. For any harsh words spoken, any unkind thoughts, like when that guy (or gal) cut you off on the freeway. It doesn't matter if you think you have nothing to forgive or be forgiven for. Try it anyway. It can't hurt. You might be surprised.

Sit or lie down in a peaceful place where you won't be disturbed for a few minutes. Breathe three times slowly and become deeply quiet... Repeat the prayer several times, slooow-ly. Let its meaning touch your heart. If an incident rises up unexpectedly, some painful memory from your past, let it be. Acknowledge it, but go back to repeating the prayer. Don't stop until you feel complete. Tears may come. If they do, let them. Letting out our emotions helps to release the energy it has taken to hold any animosity in place. Have a journal close at hand, so you can jot down any thoughts or feelings that may be revealed.

I'm sorry,
Please forgive me,
I love you,
Thank you.

When you have finished, sit quietly, allowing your body-mind to return to conscious awareness. Give yourself time to process what just took place. Pick up your journal and write about your experience. If nothing came, write that. If you think it was a waste of time, write that, but acknowledge yourself for being willing to go through the process, for acknowledging that we all make mistakes and pray to be forgiven when we do.

Throw open wide those prison doors and *run*, do not walk out into the light of a brand new day! Be grateful for the wisdom gained, the lessons learned, bless and release the "other," who is really an aspect of you in a different body.

When you have utterly and completely released the issue and everyone involved in it, you will still remember the facts, but the Energy around it will be gone. Notice if you feel lighter and have a greater sense of peace. It's best not to rush back into your day too quickly. Your To Do list can wait. Let these good feelings rest in you for a while.

Tip #4: Forgive yourself utterly and completely and waste not another precious moment of your blessed life. Give thanks and be grateful for your new-found freedom. Vow to catch yourself if you begin to wander down that old path of judgement and condemnation, replaying an old worn-out record and simply decide to make a new, happier choice.

Chapter 5

Feeling Sad, Lonely, Depressed, Scared?

"Everyone is a bit scared,
but we are less scared together."
~ Charlie Mackesy, *The Boy, The Mole, The Fox and the Horse*

When I found myself in the hospital for the fourth time with heart and lung issues, I was scared. I faced my own mortality for the first time, and it shook me to my core. Through the long, sleepless nights, my wild imagination could lead me down the dark path of doubt and fear when I let it. The feeling was so strong, I felt like I couldn't breathe. I had to *consciously choose* again and again to *turn away* from fear and doubt and *turn toward* the

Power that is greater than I am that is right where I am in every moment. My caring doctors and nurses helped me understand the changes that were taking place in my body and what I could do to help myself walk through it back to health and wholeness.

Everyone feels sad or scared at times, but what I discovered was that my *experience* was being created entirely in my own mind. If I let my thoughts sink down into fear of the future unknown, it could quickly overwhelm me. However, if I chose to hum a faith-filled song, or repeat an encouraging phrase over and over, or write my thoughts in my journal, the darkness would lift and I could smile again, trust again. That's when we most need another who can see the Truth for us when we can't see it for ourselves. We do not deny the facts, but a higher Truth is here for our taking. There is an unlimited Power, everywhere present; right where I am, right where you are in every moment. When we turn to It and call upon It in faith and trust, believing, It responds to answer our need.

Thank God, I had dear, faithful, friends and family members, who reminded me all I had to live for and the indomitable energy I've always been blessed with. They reminded me that I had a Higher Power I could call on at any time, even in the middle of the night, when the creepers of doubt and fear try to sneak in.

I volunteered for a year at the World Ministry of Prayer at Sixth Street and Vermont in Los Angeles. Every time we entered the sacred space to start our four-hour shifts, we began with this simple prayer.

Peace is the power at the heart of God

Think about it. The sun rises every day, bringing light and warmth, making life possible on planet earth. Yet there are no drum rolls, no marching bands, to herald its arrival. It does its work in silence, in perfect peace. No effort, no struggle, no blue Mondays, or holidays off. With great wisdom, it gives freely and equally to all. The birds don't vocalize to warm up their voices, they just sing for the pure joy of singing. Grass grows, fruit appears on the trees, babies are born, and the world keeps spinning.

All of life gives of itself without struggle, simply *allowing* the wisdom of Nature to lead the way. You have that same spiritual guidance system, your SGS, within you. It came with your package. You didn't do anything to earn it and you can't do anything to destroy it. It is here to serve you and me and all of creation.

Sometimes I forget the depths of the unconditional love that the Universe has for me, and I feel less than good, less than worthy. Life is a journey and just as the weather changes from day to day, so do our life experiences. When you feel sad, lonely, depressed or just plain scared, what do you do? Do you have ideas or practices in place to help shift your energy from fear back to love?

Life is this Infinite Power for Good Expressing Itself. All of life. Not just some of life, but all of it, from the song of the bird, to the shining of the sun, to the beating of our hearts, to the sweet breath that fills our lungs. How could we not be grateful? How could we not dance with joy and sing songs of praise all day long? Some days I could, and some days I couldn't, and it's all OK.

It's OK to be right where you are, feeling what you're feeling, having the experiences you're having. Talk out loud to those shadows if they come in the night. Tell them to get out! You don't want them, don't need them. They don't belong to you. They're not real. They are a figment of your own imagination. *No one thinks in your mind but you.*

Tip #1: Good news: If you created them, you can un-create them! Erase and Replace! Erase the downers and replace them with an upper. Play some music, dance in your underwear in the kitchen, (Yep! Done that one), sing out of tune, as loud as you can! Howl at the moon, bake something yummy. Give a gift to someone you would never think to give a gift to.

If you need it, physical therapy will help you get back on your feet. There are times when we just can't do it alone. We need help and it's OK to ask for and accept it. They will help you return to vibrant health and wellness. The therapists become your new best friends. I could hardly move my feet to walk when I left the hospital. I kind of shuffled along with a walker. Use one if you need it. It's only temporary. As your energy returns, you'll know when it's time to let it go and move to a cane. One year later, I haven't even needed a cane for sometime now. But in the beginning, we tend to go up and down; the hills and valleys of our life journey. Rejoice in the hills that lift you up and be gentle, kind, and patient with yourself when you find yourself in a valley.

Tip #2: Get outside! Nothing lifts your spirits like fresh air and sunshine. Eat your lunch or dinner outside. I do, every chance I get. Listen to the birds, drink in the blue sky, and let all of Nature fill you with joy and laughter. If you're lucky like me, you might hear children playing outside, near your home. Rejoice and give thanks for it. They are expressing and experiencing the pure joy of life.

Tip #3: Take a walk. Walking is the second-best exercise for our bodies, after swimming as number one. It's free and it's easy. Years ago, following a miserable back injury, I was not getting better. Having done everything the medical and chiropractic world had to offer, I said to myself, "You have to get out and walk!" The first day I could only go the length of one house and then sat down on the curb to rest. The second day I went two houses. It was easy to keep increasing the distance a little bit each day. It also gets you out of the house, where you might be feeling lonely and blue. You just might run into a neighbor who is looking for someone to talk to, someone just like you.

Tip #4: Plant something: flowers, or carrots if you're a serious gardener. I got this idea that I would grow my own food. My mom and dad did it, so I could too! Right? Wrong! I must have other talents, because a farmer I am not. I did eat a few Romain lettuce leaves in my salad before the bugs ate the rest. But I am *thrilled* when the 20+ plus pots on my patio burst into bloom with pansies, snapdragons, lavender, petunias, and more. A veritable spring garden. I have the great privilege of tending to them. I love pruning them, talking to them, welcoming the new growth, and blessing those who need to be removed to make way for something new. It has become my happy place. What's yours?

One more thing before I wrap this up. When Physical Therapy kicked me out, they said, "You're done. You don't need us anymore," I felt sad. They became my friends over the months we worked together. I had regained my strength with their help and I wanted to thank them. I baked my mother's famous Boulangerie Lemon Cake and took it to them still warm on a Friday at lunchtime when I knew they'd all be there. It gave me such joy to see the surprise and appreciation on their faces, and it warmed my heart to know I could give too.

At my last checkup, Dr Sapo listened to my heart and said, "It's in sinus (rhythm)." I believe my heart has healed itself! Thank you, God! Thank you for holding me and guiding me through the long, dark nights when I was scared and could not find my way. Thank you for the amazing nurses at Henry Mayo Hospital who loved me through my stuff and made me laugh. We shared pictures of our grandkids, and the last one hugged me when I left.

Maybe I need to bake them a lemon cake too.

The following is a list of Tips and ideas about how to have more Fun in your life! It is also a Tool to help you get out of the dumps if they ever show up. Instead of bemoaning, what you *can't* do, (If I can't Salsa...too fast) celebrate what you *can* do, (I can Rumba! Slower). So here we go! Have fun with it and create some wild and crazy suggestions of your own!

Tip# 5: Do not let yourself fall into the trap of 'I can't.' Now you can leave it saying, "Oh yes, I Can!"

TIPS & TOOLS:

Lying on the couch on and off for months following my hospital stays was a real downer. I wasn't able to go out into the world and do what I loved; going on auditions, shooting a tv show, or driving to San Diego to visit family. Every day I had to Choose between pulling myself up by the boot straps to face another day with gratitude and grace, or sulking because I couldn't go to my Latin Dance class. Some days I made it and some days not, but in learning how to live in this changed body, I discovered some Tips and Tools. So, instead of bemoaning what you *can't* do, (show up at your granddaughter's swim party in a string bikini or speedo) celebrate what you *can* do!

If you can't walk, can you sing?
If you can't sing, can you dance?
If you can't dance, can you yodel?
If you can't yodel, can you hula hoop?
If you can't hula hoop, can you teach yoga?
If you can't teach yoga, can you learn Spanish?
If you can't learn Spanish, can you knit or crochet?
If you can't knit or crochet, can you learn to swim?
If you can't learn to swim, can you create a podcast?
If you can't create a podcast, can you plant a garden?
If you can't plant a garden, can you paint a picture?
If you can't paint a picture, can you do a crossword puzzle?
If you can't do a crossword, can you learn Mah-jongg?
If you can't learn Mah-jongg, can you do pole dancing?
If you can't do pole dancing, can you volunteer?
If you can't volunteer, can you meditate?

If you can't meditate, can you play music?
If you can't play music, can you play dominoes?

<u>Your turn:</u> fill in the blanks, or pick up your journal and have at it:

If I can't _____ I can _____

If I can't _____ I can _____

A couple more inspiring ideas. Don't be afraid to write something wild like go skydiving. When we're willing to write outrageous, silly, ridiculous stuff, sometimes the really good stuff, the Real Stuff, shows up right after that. Play with it. Have fun and make it easy!

If you can't play dominoes, can you play a flute?
If you can't play a flute, can you polish your nails?
If you can't polish your nails, can you bake some cookies?
If you can't bake some cookies, can you go on a cruise?

You've got the idea. Have more inspiring ideas? Write them below, or in your journal.

_____

Chapter 6

Love Life, Love Others

*My daughter-in-law has a plaque on the wall
in her guest bathroom.
It says: Love God, Love People.*

If you can't throw your arms around God in gratitude for all the blessings in your life, you can throw your arms around your neighbor, or a friend, or a pet. We love God by loving people... who are God in disguise... just like you and me.

Made in the image and after the likeness of the Divine, you too are divine regardless of what anyone says. If you were made out of Whole Cloth, wouldn't you be Whole? And if you are made out of the fabric of the Divine, wouldn't you be divine? Shot from God, you are a beautiful, irreplaceable, unique expression of the Divine. Deep in your soul is a part of you that has never been hurt or abandoned or abused, as pure and innocent as the day you were born. That's Who You Really Are, holy and whole. It's who you were before you came into form on this earth and who you will be when you leave it.

I caught a vision early in my spiritual training regarding living and moving and having my being in the Divine, while the Divine lived and moved and had It's Being in me. It was too big for me to wrap my head around until I had this vision:

As the fish swims through the water, the water swims through the fish.

My understanding has grown from this early vision, because the water and the fish are still two separate things. But we're not separate—we are One and the same thing.

Notice how you *feel* when you are caught for a moment in the grandeur of a sunset, riot with changing colors; or a symphony, or painting, or how the sun sparkles on the oceans waves as dolphins glide side by side and you melt into the moment. That's God! That's you letting go and letting your soul soar and sing in harmony with the Divine. That's you replaying a distant memory, even if just for a moment, when you knew who you were. That's what Joseph Campbell told us to do in his book, *The Power of Myth*: *follow your bliss.*

That was you, blissing out on the shore, mesmerized by the grace with which the dolphins moved effortlessly in perfect harmony and rhythm with each other and all of Nature around them.

A few years ago, I was at a retreat that began at 7:00 AM on Zuma Beach. About twenty-five of us held hands in a circle near the water's edge while Dr James Mellon gave the opening prayer. I felt so moved by the environment, the cool breeze, the sound of the waves crashing on the shore, I opened my eyes for a moment and gazed out to sea. What I saw made me catch my breath. Two dolphins were slowly swimming from right to left, *right in front of us*, as close to the shore as possible and I knew they came to welcome us, to communicate with us. They stayed close by the whole morning and it just felt magical.

To add to the magic, later that morning a young whale joined our gathering. We could hardly believe it. It too came close to the shore, just off to our right and stayed there for hours while the playful dolphins circled it and made it welcome.

Tip#1: Remember a specific time when you forgot yourself and melted into the moment. Recreate it now. Let yourself *feel* your heart swell as the bliss of the moment engulfs you. You can recreate this feeling of bliss any time you choose, because your subconscious mind, which runs all your automatic systems continuously and faultlessly, doesn't know the difference between what's real and what's imagined. The fact that this is not a new idea doesn't diminish it's Power or availability to you.

Set aside time in your spiritual practice to recreate these feelings of bliss, of feeling your oneness with all of Life. The more you practice these precious moments, the more they will become a natural part of your experience. You are choosing to focus on the Beauty and Joy of Life instead of the daily distractions and drama. It will be easy, because it's already inside of you. As you feel gratitude well up in your heart, use that energy to bless another.

Tip #2: Write a note of appreciation to someone who helped you along the way. Someone who lifted you up when you were down and needed a friend. Do not text! Mail it.

Tip #3: Write a note of appreciation from the Universe to you, thanking you for reaching out to others in need. Let the Universe acknowledge the loving kindness, the generosity of heart and spirit with which you have blessed others when they were in need. Begin with *Dear* _____ (your name) and end with: *Love, Life.* Mail it to yourself.

Tip #4: When you receive it, Let It In! Wait until you can sit alone, quietly to open and read it. Do not fluff it off. Read it as if you have never seen it before—as if Life Itself were pouring out Its love and appreciation for you.

Tip #5: Save it. Tuck it away so that you might accidentally come across it in the future. You are made new in each moment, so the person who reads it then will not be the same person who read it earlier. You will have changed. Let it touch your heart. You may even feel like crying.

The following is a Buddhist prayer of Loving-Kindness that you might enjoy. Its purpose is to cultivate unconditional love for all. There are as many variations of this prayer as there are self-help books. I have decided to create my own version from those I've read, which is shorter than most.

> May I be happy
> May I be well
> May I be peaceful
> May I be at ease.

Repeat it slowly, meaningfully, until you feel all tension dissolve from your body/mind. When you feel 'at ease,' begin it again for others. You may have a particular person or persons in mind, but that is not necessary.

> May you be happy
> May you be well
> May you be peaceful
> May you be at ease.

Take your time. Finally speak it for the world and everyone in it.

> *May all beings be happy*
> *May all beings be well*
> *May all beings be peaceful*
> *May all beings be at ease.*

Know your simple prayer, said with conscious intention, is contributing to Peace in the world in our time.

If you're interested in learning more ways you can contribute to peace on our planet, check out *Golden Path of Peace*, by Rev. Barbara Leger. Her *Peace First* program in the Ukraine to date has reached 14,000 school age children through 198 teachers in 115 schools in the past three years. It's training tomorrow's leaders today!

Chapter 7

Want More Intimacy, Love, and Sex?

"Sexual energy, or eros, is life force
that permeates all creation and is
part of the joyfulness of life."
~ Christiane Northrup, M.D., *Women's
Bodies, Women's Wisdom*

We are not meant to live in isolated caves in the Himalayas. We are a tribal people. We need each other. Covid taught us that, especially those of us who live alone. How grateful we were, how it filled our hearts to overflowing to hug each other again. To look deeply into another's eyes to see our love for all of humanity reflected there. We were Alive. We'd gotten through it together and we were grateful.

As a celibate widow for seven years, following the unexpected death of my beloved husband of nearly fifty years, I never thought about sex. I didn't long for it or miss it, at least that's what I thought. It was as if that aspect of my life never existed. It was just gone, dead to me... until I had a blind date. My first one ever, and at the age of 75!

He had asked through friends to meet me at our favorite club, where Esther and I danced and sang the night away to the tunes of our favorite DJ. The moment he touched me, I was swept away. It had been so long since I'd been held in the arms of a warm-blooded, attractive man, it broke me wide-open. I felt the desire grow in me to love and be loved again. Although nothing ever happened between Keith and me, he brought me a great gift. He melted my broken, ice bound heart so I could love again.

Later when I met a handsome 'silver fox' in Ojai, California, that spark in my heart burst into flames. Over time we became lovers and continued to date over the next two years. I felt like a woman again, desired, and desirable. He was everything I needed in a companion, a friend, a partner, in exploring life, and each other. I learned a lot about myself. He too gave me a gift. He awakened me again to my natural sexuality and I will be forever grateful.

While our bodies change over time, our need for love and companionship does not. It may even grow stronger. When we find ourselves alone, all those treasured moments of bliss we took so for granted in our marriages or long-term relationships no longer exist.

> "Making love is one of those magical experiences when your soul manifests through your body. Time disappears and the boundaries of separateness dissolve." ~ Christian Sorenson, *Living From the Mountaintop*

I remember walking in the parking lot at Trader Joe's and seeing an older couple in front of me holding hands. I spoke to them and told them how it warmed my heart to see them holding hands and how much I missed doing that with my husband who is no longer with me. In fact, that's one of the things I missed most about our life together. It's that unspoken connection between long time lovers and partners, where no words are needed. There is a silent, heart to heart communication going on. It says, *I am here. You can count on me. I've got your back and I know you've got mine. Anything that shows up in our lives, we will tackle and overcome together.*

Intimacy begins with me, but if we can't be intimate with ourselves, how can we hope to be so with another? To me, intimacy means surrendering to the object of our love and devotion. But if we haven't accepted ourselves, if we don't love ourselves utterly and completely, with all our warts and wrinkles, we don't have a whole complete person to offer to another.

> "I can't stress enough how important it is
> to cultivate a deep love affair
> with yourself."
> ~Anita Moorjani, *Dying to Be Me*

I must admit, that sounds like an ego trip to me, but that is not the author's intent. In fact, it's just the opposite. She says in her book, what she learned from her NDE, or Near Death Experience, is that the entire Universe is made of Unconditional Love! We are *that* and couldn't be anything else! It is our nature, our very essence, but most of us were not taught that. So, I invite you to fall in love with your humanity and your divinity at the same time. Fall in love with all the ways you've tried to find love and to *be* love waiting to be found. Celebrate all the myriad ways you've succeeded, and all the ways you haven't.

Our relationships help to shape us. Bumping up against those with different points of view, different ideas of what a relationship even looks like or feels like, changes you.

As a young bride, I used to get so upset with my husband because he didn't fulfill all my *unspoken* needs, wants or desires. I obviously expected him to read my mind! His answer was always some variation of, *I thought if you needed my help you'd ask.*

My old patterns of sulking, pouting, and playing the silent game, never got me what I wanted. I had to learn to face my insecurities, those 'fears' and ask for what I wanted plain and simple. When I did, he was usually happy to fulfill it. I am still practicing that lesson out in the world as well as at home.

To me, intimacy indicates a willingness to be seen deeply all the way to your soul. No hiding, no masks, no excuses. Arguments may happen, disagreements, but these can actually clear the air and be a catalyst for deeper understanding between two partners as you come together in love. But only if you stay open hearted, willing to really listen to the other person and hear what they are courageous enough to share.

That which you are seeking is seeking you.

There is someone out there seeking exactly what you have to offer. The steps you are taking are creating a welcome space for that particular person to fill. They are not a waste of time or an excuse for not getting out there and looking for what you really want. You are preparing yourself to welcome your new beloved. Going to the gym, working out to get your body in better shape is fine, but the real work is done on the inside, in your heart and mind.

If you are single and ready to explore the possibility of finding a new partner, a new relationship, there are things you can do in the physical world to help prepare the way.

<u>Tip #1:</u> Ask yourself if you are really ready to welcome a new partner at this time. Go deep. Sit quietly and allow your feelings to reveal themselves. Are you just lonely? That could be part of it, but it may not be enough to establish a lasting relationship, if that's what you want.

<u>Tip #2:</u> Have you completely released your previous relationship with love? You will not be free to accept a new one until you do. Write a letter to that person which you won't mail. Write about the good times you shared as well as your sadness and disappointment that it's over.

<u>Tip #3</u>: *Acknowledge your part in the break-up*. It takes two to tango and two to disagree. Accepting your part allows you to heal and release it, therefore not carrying it into the next relationship. Your ego hates this part. Do it honestly, asking to be shown what you could do better next time, then release it all with love. End with gratitude for all the things you learned while you were together. Then set them

free with your blessing, wishing them the best. Since we are all one in consciousness, you can't want something for yourself that you deny to another. In your heart, want the best for All!

Tip #4: If you are in a committed long-term relationship, Rev. Marilyn Miller suggests scheduling a weekly sit-down together, to discuss anything that needs your attention; any doubts, concerns, hopes or dreams. Set a time limit, say 30 minutes. Just get it out. Nothing can be resolved unless you are willing to discuss it. It may be messy, but that's OK. Talking out little issues before they become mountains of resentment or resistance is way easier than letting them ferment over time. Keep it light. Take a moment before you start to remind each other how much you love one another. You might even mention one specific thing they did that week that you appreciated and forgot to thank them for.

Tip #5: Another person can't complete you. You are not half of anything. You are already whole and complete, a vibrant expression of the divine, ready to share your heart, soul and possibly home, with another. If you hear yourself say, *I'll only be happy when....* , you are heading down the wrong road. Detour! Actually, the reverse is true. When you are truly happy *First,* grateful and open to life's adventures, your energy will be so attracting, you won't be able to keep your dream partner away!!!

Tip #6: Walk through your home with the eyes of a stranger. Does it look and feel ready to welcome a special guest? If you were throwing a party, you'd have a long list of things you'd want to accomplish before they arrived. Do those things.

Are your bathroom towels the ones that you got for a wedding gift years ago? Buy new ones. Clean your closet. Give things away. Make physical space for this new exciting adventure to begin. It may be down the road a piece, but you are acting as if it's already *here, now*.

You get the idea. To wrap this up, I thought it would be fun to add a few comments from some of my favorite, single, senior friends. Take it from me, they are awesome!

J., 80 years young in Westlake California writes:
"I love life! I am definitely open to a loving, caring, romantic relationship that includes friendship, and support as well as sex. We have each other's backs. I have had wonderful relationships and relationships that were not so wonderful, but they were the exception, not the rule."

M., 74 years young, in Santa Clarita, California says this:
"I want a casual relationship leading to a commitment of sorts. I don't know what a sexual relationship looks like at this age, or if I even want one. These are the 4C's that are absolute for me: Chemistry, Compatibility, Com-

munication, Commitment. On these I will not compromise."

M., 80 years young, Ojai, California writes:
"I have been married three times, divorced twice, and widowed once. I have decided to spare what's left of the senior male population in Southern California and remain single."

E., 74 years young, Encinitas, California writes in caps:
"MY DESIRE IN A RELATIONSHIP IS INTIMACY: IN-TO-ME-I-SEE. When I am willing to see, accept and share the love and beauty in me, I will be prepared to accept that special person's love."

S., 74 years young, Kauai, Hawaii writes:
"The truth is, I just won't settle for a relationship that doesn't make my heart sing."

On reading this chapter, one of our mutual male friends commented:
"Do not do 'One and Done!' Mix and Mingle. GET OUT THERE!"

Chapter 8

Your Turn: Take Action

A 4 Week Plan to Live Your Best Life at Any Age

That buzz of excitement when you discover something new and life changing is fleeting. How to *sustain it over time*, that's our task, our next step. Decide when you will begin, count ahead and mark 4 weeks on your calendar, circling the end date.

WEEK ONE

At the beginning of the week, read the book again. It should take about one hour.

After reading through the book, choose one thing that jumps out at you: relationships, forgiveness, get moving again etc. Write it at the top of a page in your journal. Write any specific person or situation that came up for you if it did, but that is not necessary. Next, write the *Changed Experience* you desire to see in this situation.

Now that you've done that, for the rest of the week, set aside 15 minutes each day to work on your chosen topic.

Follow the prompts in the chapter: write an affirmation, repeat the prayers, journal. Write any insights that come to you as you do your work each day, including any '*Changes in the Experience*' you are starting to see.

Congratulate yourself on your willingness to set aside this special time just for you.

WEEK TWO

Review the previous week: What did you learn? What surprised or delighted you? What changed? Did you take any risks? Did you do that scary thing? Write it in your journal.

Next, pick another topic that interests you, and repeat the week one process for that topic.

Now you're two weeks into the review, and you've done meaningful work on two important topics that matter to you.

WEEK THREE

Repeat Week Two, choosing another topic to work with.

Write a positive, present-tense statement relating to your topic. Put it in your phone and refer to it throughout the day. Keep it short, clear and full of emotion, which is 'energy in motion!' Put the Power of your Intention into it. Repeat it aloud with meaning several times a day, especially just before falling asleep and immediately upon waking up.

WEEK FOUR

Repeat Week Three, choosing another topic. If you find yourself strongly resisting any particular topic, know that's where the greatest opportunity for growth lies for you.

Congratulations! You completed the 4 Week Plan and are richer for it. Having done the work, be sure to write your *'Changed Experience'* in your journal. Write how you *feel* about the changes for the better you are making.

You'll notice that you have now done a deep dive on four of the book's seven chapters. If you are inspired to keep going, have at it!

Reward Yourself! Because you deserve it! Ask yourself what would make you feel special, pampered, cared for and loved. Because you are, far more than you will ever know.

Well, my friends, we have come to the end of our journey together, however, it needn't end. You can continue repeating the process, choosing a different topic each week. You may even decide to go back and do more work on an earlier topic you chose.

Now you know how this 'Thinking Stuff' works and how you can cooperate with it to live your Best Life at Any Age! The Truth is, you knew it all along. It was all already inside of you just waiting for you to come out and Play!

And before we say goodbye for now, I'd like to invite you to keep the conversation going. If you have your own stories of living your best life at any age, I'd love to hear from you! Please reach out at:

NancyB-FreetoBe.com
Instagram: nberggren16
Facebook: Nancy B. Berggren

I AIN'T DEAD YET
Music and Lyrics by Nancy B. Berggren

Gramma's right happy and doin' just fine,
Kick up my heels, swillin' cheap wine.
Done fooled 'em all, those fancy pants docs.
Cain't shut love in an old pine box.

I got a smile on my face or down on my luck,
I'm rollin in dough or can't make a buck.
But listen real close, 'cause I'm telling you true,
Here's what happened and the jokes on you.

Git out the way, git offa my back,
I'm on the move, I'm on the right track.
Git out the way, cuz you can bet,
I'm on the move, and I ain't dead yet.

So, call off the diggers, send the hearse home,
There'll be no Wake, Gramma's commin' home.
Let's have a party, a real shivareee.
I'll keep on dancin' while I can still breathe.

Git out the fiddle and resin up the bow,
Beat out the time while we do-sa-do.
I ain't kicked the bucket, least not yet.
Call off the Wake 'cause I ain't dead yet.

Git out the way, git offa my back,
I'm on the move, I'm on the right track.
Git out the way, cuz you can bet,
I'm on the move and I ain't dead yet.

Acknowledgements

My heartfelt thanks to Thor Challgren for creating his *Your Book Now* class in which this book was written. He takes what seems overwhelming and makes it easy, by breaking it down into bite sized chunks. He also held my hand and guided me through the process that takes place *after* the writing is done! Thank you, Thor!

To all my inspiring teachers and mentors along the way. But especially Dr. James Mellon, founder of the Global Truth Center in Westlake, who took me in after I retired from the Fallbrook Center for Spiritual Living, where I was the senior minister for ten years. The Revs. Brian Anderson, Dr. Christian Sorenson, Dr. Linda McNamar, and Michael Reiss; my coaches, friends, and mentors and who I turn to for inspiration regularly. Richest blessings.

To my prayer partners and BFF's who dance with me when I'm up and lift me up when I'm down: Esther Jones, Marilyn Taylor, Sue Wood, Rev. Marilyn Miller, Dona Oxford, Rev. Barbara Leger and Rev. Hilde Brooks. Each and every one of you are the inspiration that filled every word in this book. You are my shining light, my strong survivors, my truth-tellers, my 'encouragers' and my dearest friends.

Last but not least: the brilliant Dr. Lori Savage who created the Fabulous Cover!!! Couldn't have done it without you.

Finally, to my big, amazing, talented, brilliant, ever-growing family who have loved me, and are always there for me, no matter what, through all my ups and downs. Most especially, my four wonderful kids; Steve Berggren, Lisa Berggren, Linda Donais and Scott Berggren. We don't always agree, but we always know, deep down, that love heals all things and that family is *Everything*.

Books That Changed My Life

Here are a few books that have brought meaning to my life.

Living From the Mountaintop, Christian Sorenson
The Power of Decision, Raymond Charles Barker
Meditation for Daily Stress, Michel Pascal
This Thing Called You, Ernest Holmes
Breaking the Habit of Being Yourself, Dr. Joe Dispenza
Proof of Heaven, Eben Alexander, M.D.
The Holy Bible, King James Version
The Abundance Book, John Randolph Price
The Artists Way, Julia Cameron

About the Author

At 91 years young, Nancy B. pours her passion and love of life into everything she does. She is a dynamic and inspiring international speaker, published author, actor, non-denominational minister, and proud grandmother of 24 grand and great-grandchildren!

Nancy B is blessed to have worked recently opposite *Jim Carrey* in *Kidding*; in *Rutherford Falls*, *Shining Vale*, *iCarly,* in the feature film, *Bromates* and at the famous *Comedy Store* in Hollywood: and all in her late 80's!

For guest speaking and book signing opportunities:

NancyB-FreetoBe.com
Instagram:nberggren16
Facebook: Nancy B. Berggren

Made in the USA
Columbia, SC
02 July 2024